Create A Miracle
With Hexagonal Water

The Simple Solution For Vital Health And Longevity

Dr. Howard Peiper, N.D.

Create a Miracle
With Hexagonal Water

by
Dr. Howard Peiper N.D.

Copyright © 2008 by Dr. Howard Peiper, edited by Nina Anderson

All Rights Reserved

No part of this book may be reproduced in any form
without the written consent of the publisher.

ISBN 1-884820-91-3
ISBN 13: 978-1-884820915
Library of Congress Catalog Card Number 2008929310

Printed in the United States of America

Create a Miracle with Hexagonal Water is not intended as medical advice. It is written solely for informational and educational purposes. Please consult a health professional should the need for one be indicated. Because there is always some risk involved, the author and publisher are not responsible for any adverse effects or consequences resulting from the use of any of the suggestions, preparations or methods described in this book. The publisher does not advocate the use of any particular diet or health program, but believes the information presented in this book should be made available to the public.

Published by
ATN Publishing
561 Shunpike Rd.
Sheffield MA 01257
www.longlifecatalog.com
888-628-8731

Preface

Humans have survived for as many as ninety days without food, but can live only seventy-two hours without water before going into a semi-comatose state. However, drinking water saturated with inorganic minerals such as magnesium carbonate, calcium carbonate and other elements the body cannot use, may lead to a variety of unhealthy conditions. These inorganic minerals, toxic chemicals, fluoride and other contaminants can pollute, clog up and even turn tissues to stone throughout our body, causing pain, illness and even premature death. Hexagonal water, nature's healing water, helps remove inorganic mineral deposits and toxins from the joints, may remove cholesterol and fat, and creates a pH balance in our body. This book unlocks the mysteries of hexagonal water, which can relieve chronic suffering. Using the miracle of hexagonal water has been proven to help us live healthier and longer lives.

Howard Peiper N.D.

Table of Contents

Chapter 1	Solved, The Secret Mystery of Aging!	7
Chapter 2	Acidity – The Grim Reaper!	9
Chapter 3	Alkalinity Conquers Death	13
Chapter 4	Dehydration – Am I Thirsty?	15
Chapter 5	pH and Cellular Health	19
Chapter 6	Weight Gain, High Blood Pressure and Cholesterol	25
Chapter 7	Rheumatoid Arthritis Pain	27
Chapter 8	Cellular Oxygen Deficiency and Cancer	29
Chapter 9	So, What's In Your Water?	31
Chapter 10	Sports Drinks and Bottled Water	35
Chapter 11	What in the World is Hexagonal Water?	39
Chapter 12	The Kangen™ Water Experience	45
Chapter 13	What People are Saying	51
	Resources	57
	Bibliography	59
	About The Author	61

Chapter One

"Physicians think they are doing something for us by labeling what we have as a disease"
Immanuel Kant

Solved, The Secret Mystery of Aging!

We are programmed to get old and look old, but it doesn't have to be that way. Age and longevity are relative. Some people at age 65 look 45 – others at 65 look 85.

Nobody denies genes. Our parents have an awful lot to do with our physical and mental makeup. But we can do a great deal to improve our looks and our quality of life. Aging without quality of life is not exciting. We can make a big difference, but only if we believe that we can, and then take action.

First and most important is to know what we put in our mouth. Americans are starving to death. Yes, we are consuming larger and larger amounts of "food", getting fatter and fatter, and sicker and sicker. Nobody is enjoying this except the medical establishment. There are plenty of sick people.

Here is what's happening. We are consuming tasty foods (so-called) that have calories and produce energy but lack nutrition. Did you know that some foods have calories that produce energy but have no nutrition? This is the definition of the beautifully packaged commercial foods that we eat. In fact, this is mostly what Americans consume and we gradually starve to death. Empty foods as described above not only do not provide nutrition, they build and accumulate as toxemia or poison in the body and in the blood. The accumulation of toxins in the body is the beginning of death. Death is the result of toxemia. Diseases and death is a common expression of toxemia.

Think, now! Disease cannot be its own cause; neither can it be its own cure – and certainly not its own prevention. We cause disease ourselves. Sickness and low quality of life go hand in hand. There is no life or vitality in antibiotics or flu shots or immunization. Life, beauty and youth are in the blood and good blood is made of good food.

Good blood, vigorous health and stamina cannot come from a subsistence on white bread, doughnuts, pies, cakes, latte's and pretty packaged commercial foods sold at the supermarket. Consider all the tens of thousands of preparations including most so-called "health foods" and cereals. Include all the "food" that has been dyed or treated chemically to have a beautiful appearance, fried, impaired and impoverished foods, pasteurized and dead foods.

The main causes of aging and disease are to be found in the derangement of normal processes of cell metabolism and cell regeneration. The accumulation of toxins (acidic foods) and metabolic waste products interferes with the nourishment of the cells and slows down cell regeneration and new cell building. When normal metabolic processes become deranged (due to nutritional deficiencies, sluggish digestion and elimination, sedentary life and overeating), and the process of cell nourishment, replacement and rebuilding slows down, our body starts to grow old. Its resistance to disease will diminish and various ills will start to appear.

Beauty, strength, youthfulness and long life occur because we select the right foods to put in our bodies. It all sounds so simple, but is it? Food is not necessarily *food*.

Chapter Two

"There is no natural death. All deaths from so-called natural causes are merely the end point of a progressive acid saturation."
Dr. George W. Crile

Acidity – The Grim Reaper!

It is not generally known that acidity (acid foods) is the principal cause of most disease.

The accumulation of acidity (acid) in the blood and the cells is the principal cause of disease and death. Leading researchers have found that there is no natural death. All deaths from so-called natural causes are merely the end points of a progressive acid saturation (toxemia).

Most of all the foods we eat are acid forming. There are so many that we cannot name them all. Almost all processed food products are acid forming. Most bottled goods are acid forming. Fats, oils (modern cooking oils), sugars, sweets, syrups, candies, starches, baked goods, cereals, glucose, jams, and jellies are acid forming. Nearly all cooked, fried and baked foods are acid forming. Almost all drugs, pills, patent medicines, drinks, tonics, wine, liquors, coffee, tea, chocolate, cocoa, and all manufactured foods are acid forming. All canned fruits almost without exception, are acid forming. Some types of canned fruit are not originally acid forming, but they become acid forming by processing; i.e., peeling, paring, cooking sweetening, preserving, or by altering and disorganizing the fruit and fruit molecules such as microwave cooking and steaming and destroying the vitamins of life. All nuts are acid forming except almonds. Most peppers and pickles are acid.

The end product of our own metabolism (catabolism) is acid forming. The products of combustion or oxidation in the body are acid forming. The dying leukocytes, dying tissues, the excreta in the bowels, the mucus, phlegm, dying bacteria, and their toxins are all acid forming. Even brain activity, thinking, worry, temper, and all sorts of unfavorable emotions result in acidity. Acidity is the father of disease.

Acid is the cause of gas generation, bloating, dullness, poor memory and low energy. So as long as we can keep the tissues nourished and keep the secretions, stomach, blood and bones alkaline, we are healthy, youthful, vigorous, efficient, lively and strong.

It is impossible to get sick so long as the human body is alkaline. It is equally impossible to keep well when the system is in an acid condition. Human alkalinity and longevity go hand in hand. Human acidity leads to disease, operations and an early funeral. An alkaline diet results in health, longevity, youth and beauty.

There is no escape from wrong choices. If we live on acid-forming foods meal after meal, year after year our body must pay the bill over and over again. Acid forming foods accumulate as toxemia. Death results from toxemia. If we must eat, we may just as well eat right. Acidity is the foundation of most of our disease, trouble, misery, pain and tears. Acidity is toxemia. Toxemia is death.

Acid in or around the nerves results in neuralgia, neuritis, sciatica, nervousness, nerve pain, headache, earache, or various nerve ailments and diseases. Acid brain matter results in inflammation of the brain, insanity, crime, violent passion, melancholia, and hundreds of symptoms of mental disease. An acid brain cannot function normally.

Acid causes arthritis, urinary ailments, heart valve problems, and kidney problems. Acidity in or around the prostate gland causes enlargement of the prostate gland, swelling and hardening, resulting in prostate cancer or at least urinary difficulties. An acid uterus leads to female complications of the menstrual cycle, inflammation, uterine tumors, and other ailments of the generative organs.

An acid liver is a disordered liver and this may result in stubborn constipation, piles, varicosis, toxicosis, auto-intoxication, hepatitis, gallstones, cirrhosis of the liver, and even insanity. The acid accumulation destroys the toxilytic functions of the liver leaving autotoxins, blood toxins, bacterial toxins, and other poisons in the blood to be carried to the brain and kidneys.

Acidity in the stomach causes gastritis, heartburn and burning in the chest. Acidity causes gas generation and gas pressure upon the heart, diaphragm, spine and other organs. Gas pressure leads to dilation of the stomach until the stomach hangs like an empty, lifeless bag, resulting in falling of the stomach, bloating, colic, indigestion, cramps, and constipation. Do we see any bloated bellies in America today?

People who are waking up are taking responsibility for their own health. They are beginning to realize that the medical establishment is dependent on its human victims for its profits.

Different diets have their effects on health and disease, but acidity is the most prolific cause of disease. One chemical body type is subject to one kind of acidity, and another type is subject to another kind of acidity and gas formation.

There are many kinds of acid responses depending on the biochemistry of the individual. The most important thing to do first is to learn what is an acid food and what is an alkaline food. Human alkalinity and longevity go hand in hand.

Seldom does a doctor in America suspect that bad diet is the cause of degenerative disease. And few would suspect that the prevailing high acid diet of Americans is the root cause of early death and suffering.

The soil in America is now so poor and so poisoned with chemical fertilizers that it is nearly impossible to buy nutritious food. The only thing left for those concerned is to get the proper whole food supplement complexes (particularly organic foods) prepared and marketed by people who are knowledgeable in human health and nutrition, and to drink alkalized, filtered water.

Chapter Three

> *"Mother Nature is man's teacher. She unfolds her treasure to his search, unseals his eyes, illuminates his mind and purifies his heart."*
> Dr. Bernard Jensen

Alkalinity Conquers Death

As we grow older, it is ever more important to know the properties of food so that we make selections that are alkaline. There is always danger of acid formation and gas generation as we live longer. Poor elimination, low vitality, tissue acidity, and autointoxication all come with age because of our ignorance of acid and alkaline foods.

Health must be developed from the inside. Beauty and youthfulness are the result of a correct alkaline diet. Grace in movement, elasticity in our arteries and tendons, and joy in living are all born of a proper diet.

When we are alkalized/balanced, there is no acidity, no gas, no autotoxins, no poisons and no accumulation of toxemia. Oxygen is abundantly supplied, the brain and nerves are well nourished, and the red blood flows vigorously to all parts of the body. Then we have regained youth and enjoy a great quality of life. We can help speed up this process by drinking alkalized water as a daily routine.

Aging may be reversed by changing our diet provided we begin before we are 90 percent dead. Aging is a disease of diet, and more specifically aging is a disease of progressive acid saturation. Because we are programmed to grow old and die does not mean that it is natural. Alkalized water can help stop this deterioration!

Acid-Forming Foods

Acid-forming foods which should be temporarily eschewed or drastically limited during the alkalinization period are principally meat, fish, poultry, eggs, cheese, fats, white bread, starchy foods, cakes, pastry, candy, white sugar, and confections. These foods are not necessarily bad but should never be taken in proportions that exceed the requirement for body need.

Alkaline Foods
(80% of diet)

Celery	Apples	Potatoes
Bananas	Carrots	Citrus fruits
Cabbage	Beets	Lettuce
Cucumbers	Asparagus	Melons
Tomatoes	Raisins	Green Beans
Pineapples	Squash	Grapes
Parsnips	Pears	Almonds
Buttermilk	Beans	Peaches
Spinach	Fresh Peas	

Acid Foods
(20% or less of diet)

Meat	Rice (polished)	Fish
Corn (dried)	Poultry	Crackers
Cheese	Hydrogenated oil	Eggs
Nuts*	Cereal	Spaghetti
Bread	White Flour	Refined
Sugar	Chocolate	Candy
Coffee/Tea	Pastry	Alcohol

Chapter Four

"The doctor of the future will give little medicine, but will interest his patients in the care of the human frame, diet, and in the cause and prevention of disease."
Thomas A. Edison

Dehydration - Am I Thirsty?

Did you know that 50-75 percent of Americans are chronically dehydrated and many of those individuals are drinking eight glasses of water a day?

Dehydration is a condition that occurs when a person loses more fluid than they take in. However, the problem is not just a lack of water, it is a lack of cellular water!

Every function of the body is monitored and pegged to the efficient flow of water. "Water distribution" is the only way of making sure that not only an adequate amount of water but also its transported elements (hormones, chemical messengers and nutrients) reach the more vital organs first. In turn, every organ that produces a substance to be made available to the rest of the body will monitor its own rate of production and release this substance into the "flowing water," according to constantly changing quotas set by the brain. Once the water itself reaches the "drier" areas it also exercises its many other vital physical and chemical regulatory actions.

Water intake and its priority distribution achieve paramount importance. The regulating neurotransmitter systems (histamine and its subordinate agents) become increasingly active during the regulation of water requirements of the body.

Water Intake and Thirst Sensations

There are basically three stages to water regulation of the body in the different phases of life. One: the stage of life of a fetus in the uterus of the mother. Interestingly when the very first indicator for water needs of the fetus appear the mother seems to get morning sickness during the early phase of pregnancy. Two: the phase of growth to adulthood. Three: the phase of growth to the demise of the person. Because of a gradually failing thirst sensation our body becomes chronically and increasingly dehydrated, starting from the early adult stage.

With increase in age the water content of the cells of the body decrease to the point that the ratio of the volume of body water inside the cells to that which is outside the cells, changes from 1.2 to 0.9. This is a drastic change. Since the "water" we drink provides the cell function and its volume requirements, the decrease in our daily water intake affects the efficiency of cell activity. It is the reason for the loss of water volume held inside the cells of the body. As a result, chronic dehydration causes symptoms that mimic disease, especially when we don't recognize the fact that we are dehydrated.

The human body can become dehydrated even when abundant water is readily available. We seem to lose our thirst sensation and the critical perception of needing water. Not recognizing our water need we become gradually, increasingly, and chronically dehydrated with progress in age. Further confusion lies in the idea that when we're thirsty, many of us often substitute tea, coffee, or alcohol-containing beverages.

The "dry mouth" is the very last sign of dehydration. The body can suffer from dehydration even when the mouth may be fairly moist. Still worse, in the elderly the mouth can be seen to be obviously dry and yet thirst may not be acknowledged and satisfied.

The best times to drink water are: one glass half-hour before eating food – breakfast, lunch, and dinner – and the same amount two hours or more after each meal. This is the very minimum amount of water our body needs. If needed, two more glasses of water should be taken around the heaviest meal or before going to bed.

Do not forget that at each phase of life, our body is the product of time-operated series of chemical interactions. It is very possible to reverse some reactions. We need not to "drown" ourselves in water. The cells of the body are like sponges; it takes some time before they become better hydrated. Also do not forget that some of them make their membranes less permissive of water diffusion, in or out.

Color of Urine
The normal color of urine should not be dark. It should ideally be almost colorless to light yellow. If it begins to become dark yellow, or even orange in color, we are becoming dehydrated. It means the kidneys are working hard to get rid of toxins in the body in very concentrated urine. That is why urine becomes darker in color. Dark color urine is a good sign of dehydration.

Chapter Five

> *"The natural healing force within us is the greatest force in getting well."*
> Hippocrates, Father of Medicine

pH and Cellular Health

The abbreviation pH stands for the power of hydrogen. A pH test using a piece of litmus paper actually measures the concentration of positively charged hydrogen ions in our body. Ions are electrically charged atoms or groups of atoms that together make up the electrical "juice" or current our body uses to communicate. The more positively-charged hydrogen ions are present, the more acidity is present. The fewer hydrogen ions are present, the less acidity. The total pH scale ranges from one to fourteen, with seven considered neutral. Anything below seven is considerate acidic and anything above seven is considered alkaline.

A healthy body functions best when it is slightly alkaline. Deviations in the blood above or below a pH range of 7.30-7.45 can signal potentially serious and dangerous symptoms of diseases. When our cell and tissue pH levels deviate from a healthy range (7.2-7.5) into an acidic state (below 7.0), the acid wastes normally back up, as in a clogged sewage system.

The pH of our blood, tissues, and bodily fluids affects the state of our cellular health and internal cleanliness. When our pH levels are in proper balance, we will experience a high degree of health and wellbeing. Every metabolic and organ/system function depends entirely on our delicately balanced pH, including all regulatory mechanisms such as digestion, metabolism, respiration, hormone release, neurotransmitter release, and immunity.

It is important to understand that the pH of our blood is critical to our lives, and to our very survival. The pH of blood has a very small degree of tolerance for variation. Our body does everything in its power to keep the pH of our blood within this neutral range, between 7.30-7.45, including pulling alkalizing minerals such as calcium out our bones and other body stores, if necessary.

If the body is overwhelmed by excess acids from poor diet or over-exposure to chemical and environmental toxins, built-in compensating mechanisms go into effect in an attempt to neutralize and excrete acidic toxins from the blood, cells, lymph, and tissue fluids. There are eight internal buffering systems the body uses to neutralize acids and balance pH. If these eight neutralizing mechanisms become overwhelmed and cannot function adequately, the excess acids will severely compromise cellular integrity and function, eventually causing a complete metabolic and system breakdown where serious health problems such as cancer may manifest.

We live and die at the cellular level. All the cells (billions of them) that make up the human body are slightly alkaline and must maintain alkalinity in order to function and remain healthy and alive. However their cellular activity creates acid and this acid is what gives the cell energy and function. As each alkaline cell performs its task of respiration it secretes metabolic wastes, and these end products of cellular metabolism are acid in nature.

Although these wastes are used for energy and function, they must not be allowed to build up. One example of this is the often painful lactic acid which is created through exercise. The body will go to any lengths to neutralize and detoxify these acids before they act as poisons in and around the cell, ultimately changing the environment of the cell. Most people and clinical practitioners believe the immune system is the body's first line of defense, but actually it is not. It is very important, but more like a very sophisticated clean-up service. We must instead look at the importance of pH balance as the first and major line of defense against sickness and disease and for health and vitality.

If we were to ask, "what is killing us," the answer might be "acidosis". Research has shown that an acidic, anaerobic (lacking oxygen) body environment encourages the breeding of fungus, mold, bacteria, and viruses. A state of acidosis is simply the lack of oxygen and available calcium, which the body uses to maintain its alkaline balance. Calcium makes up 1.5 percent of our body weight. It is literally the human glue that holds the body together. A calcium ion can hold onto six other molecules while it grabs onto one molecule of water. No other ion can do this. And it does this by taking a chain of nutrients into the cell and then leaves it to get more nutrients.

The biggest problem scientists have found is that over time the human body becomes depleted of calcium. A compound called mono-ortho-calcium phosphate is the chemical buffer for the blood. This buffer maintains the alkaline level (or the lack of acidity) in our blood. Without it we would die. If the acidity level in our blood changes even slightly we die immediately. But in order to supply enough calcium for buffering we must have enough calcium being absorbed from our diet or our body will simply extract the needed calcium from our bones and teeth.

The more acidic we become, the harder it is for oxygen to be present. Therefore, our biological terrain (inside our body) also becomes anaerobic. Without adequate oxygenation unfriendly bacteria, molds, viruses, and fungus can live and prosper. Our cells cannot carry on their life-giving functions in an efficient manner because our biological chemical reactions need oxygen.

The human body is very intelligent. As we become more and more acidic the body starts to set up defense mechanisms to keep the damaging acid from entering our vital organs. Acid gets stored in fat cells. If the acid does come into contact with an organ, the acid has a chance literally to eat holes in the tissue. This may cause cells to mutate. The oxygen level drops in this acidic environment and calcium begins to be depleted. So as a defense mechanism our body may actually make fat to protect us from our overly acidic self. Those fat cells and cellulite deposits may actually be packing up the acid and trying to keep it a safe distance from our organs. The fat may be saving our vital organs from damage. Many people have found that a return to health helps them to lose the excess fat.

Osteoporosis is very confusing for many people. Most people think they can eliminate it by increasing their consumption of milk and dairy products. But in countries where the consumption of dairy products is low the instances of osteoporosis is rare. Osteoporosis is an acidosis problem. As the body becomes more acidic, to protect against the event of heart attack, stroke, illness, or even cancer, the body attempts to remain healthy. So, it steals calcium from the bones, teeth, and tissue. As bone mass becomes depleted, this is what we call osteoporosis. As we saturate the body with calcium this brings the alkaline pH up (and drops the acid levels).

One of the first warning signs of being too acidic is the appearance of calcium deposits. A little known fact is that there has never been a scientifically proven association between calcium deposits in the body and nutritional calcium. In fact, quite the opposite is found in the results of testing calcium deposits of the body. Calcium deposits come not from dietary calcium but from the structural calcium of our bones and teeth!

When the body is overwhelmed by acidosis-toxicity, mechanisms are triggered to help neutralize the build up of poisonous acids in order to maintain a healthy, alkaline pH. Alkaline solutions (pH over 7.0) tend to absorb oxygen, while acids (pH under 7.0) tend to expel oxygen. For example, a mild alkali can absorb over 100 times as much oxygen as a mild acid. So it's a two-way street. The more acid in the body, the less ability the body fluids have to absorb oxygen. This is the classic spiral downward into disease. The more oxygen in the body, the more ability its fluid has to absorb oxygen. This is the upward spiral of health.

The first thing the body does to fight acidity is take in more oxygen the only way it knows how – through breathing harder so it can push more CO_2 out of the lungs and make room for more oxygen in the blood. Almost everyone wants more energy. How many people get winded and pant easily with a minimum of effort expended. That's low oxygen and over-acid condition plainly expressing itself when there isn't enough oxygen.

In low-oxygen cellular environments, excess carbon dioxide (carbonic acid) and lactic acid collect, so the body oxygen and intra-cellular amino acids are used up trying to buffer these acids. Lymph and saliva try to neutralize and dilute the acids, but they each thicken more as we dehydrate – thereby lowering their efficiency.

Next, our high pH electrolytes (calcium, magnesium, sodium, and potassium) are used up binding salt acids. Then our skin, urinary tract, colon and respiratory system become overloaded trying to filter them out. Then blood plasma changes while loading with bicarbonate in an attempt to neutralize the increasing acidity. If the low oxygen and minerals and water conditions persist and no change in oxygen levels, diet, or elimination are forthcoming, then the bones, teeth, joints and muscles will be robbed of their calcium, magnesium, sodium, and potassium reserves. This causes severe mineral deficiency. And, when all this fails (because the acidic mucoid sludge continues to block everything and pile up) then the body pushes the excess acids and toxins away from the core and out to be stored in the peripheral vital areas of the skin and extremities.

Diseases Related Emergency Peripheral Toxin Storage

- Acid and toxins in the wrist: carpal tunnel syndrome
- Acid and toxins in the knees: osteoarthritis
- Acid and toxins in the feet and toes: gout
- Acid and toxins in the skin: dermatitis and eczema
- Acid and toxins in the joints: rheumatoid arthritis
- Acid and toxins in the tissue: fibromyalgia, chronic fatigue, and degenerative disease, etc., etc.
- Acid and toxins in the vital organs: cancer, heart disease and serious arthritis.

The Intelligence of Cell Health

Our genetic script runs the liver's molecular machinery to store and release sugar molecules, synthesize cholesterol, detoxify the blood, secrete bile and digest hemoglobin pigment. This works in tandem with the colon cells that are simultaneously fermenting aerobic bacteria, absorbing fluid, and moving your breakfast through the intestinal tract.

Each of our molecules is a delicate instrument producing a flurry of electrochemical impulses organized by ranks of molecular switches. These turn on and off at certain intervals when necessary. A healthy body depends upon a high level of negative electromagnetic charge on tissue cells' surfaces. Acidity generates a positive charge that dampens out these electrical fields, affecting cellular communication. Unless a treatment actually removes acid toxins from the body and increases oxygen, water, and nutrients, the cure at best will only be temporary. Otherwise, the disease is driven deeper into a chronic state. The only way to properly treat disease conditions is to alkalize the pH which will dispose acids from our cells, tissues, and organs.

Chapter Six

"The body and mind are so closely connected that not even a single word or thought can come into existence without being reflected in the personality and health of the individual."
John Prentiss

Weight Gain, High Blood Pressure and Cholesterol

The central control system in the brain happens to recognize the low energy levels available for its functions. The sensations of thirst or hunger also stems from low, ready to access energy levels. To mobilize energy from that which is stored in the fat we need our hormonal release mechanisms. This process takes a while longer than the urgent needs of the brain. The front of the brain either gets energy from "hydroelectricity" or from sugar in blood circulation. Its functional needs for hydroelectricity are more urgent – not only the energy formation from water, but also its transport system within the microstream flow system that depends on more water.

The sensation of thirst and hunger are generated simultaneously to indicate the brain's needs. We do not recognize the sensation of thirst and assume "both indicators" to be the urge to eat. We eat food even when the body needs to receive water. Drinking water before eating food helps to separate the two sensations. Therefore, we are able to eat less.

High blood pressure (essential hypertension) is the result of an adaptive process to a gross body water deficiency. When we do not drink enough water to serve all the needs of the body some cells become dehydrated and lose some of their water to the circulation. Capillary beds in some areas will have to close so that some of the slack in capacity is adjusted for. In water shortage and body drought, 66 percent is lost from water held in the cells, 27 percent is taken from water volume held outside the cells, and 7 percent is taken from blood volume. The blood cells then close lumen (void space just inside the cell wall) to compensate for the water loss, causing hypertension. Therefore, the major cause for blood volume loss is the loss of body water or its undersupply through the loss of thirst sensation – and when we lose thirst sensation (or do not recognize signals of hydration) and drink less water than the daily requirement, the shutting down of some vascular beds is the only natural alternative to keep the rest of the blood vessels full.

When diuretics are administered to remove excess water, the body becomes more dehydrated. The "dry mouth" from dehydration is reached and some water is taken to compensate. Diuretics cannot solve the problem of water retention because it is caused by dehydration.

Higher blood cholesterol is a sign that the cells of the body have developed a defense mechanism against the osmotic force of the blood that keeps drawing water out through the cell membranes to maintain normal cell function. Cholesterol production in the cell membrane is a part of the cell survival system. It is a necessary substance. Its excess denotes dehydration.

In a well-hydrated cell membrane, water is the adhesive material that also diffuses through the hydrocarbon "bricks". The bilayer is separated and the space is used as a "waterway" for enzyme activity. In a dehydrated cell membrane cholesterol is manufactured to stick the "bricks" together and also prevents further loss of water from inside the cell. If we drink water before we eat food, the battle against cholesterol formation in the blood can be won.

Chapter Seven

"Water is the essential fluid of all life, the solvent of our ills and can be the deliverer of a radiant, healthy, long life."
Masaru Emoto

Rheumatoid Arthritis Pain

Over 60 million Americans suffer from some form of arthritis, 30 million people suffer from low back pain, millions suffer from arthritic neck pains, and over 300,000 children are affected by the juvenile form of arthritis. Once any of these conditions establishes in an individual it becomes a sentence to suffering.

Rheumatoid arthritic joints and their pain are to be viewed as indicators of water deficiency in the affected joint cartilage surfaces. Arthritis pain is another of the regional thirst signals of the body.

The cartilage surfaces of bones in a joint contain much water. The lubricating property of this "held water" is utilized in the cartilage allowing the two opposing surfaces to freely glide over one another during joint movement.

The bone cells are immersed in calcium deposits and the cartilage cells are immersed in a matrix containing much water. As the cartilage surfaces glide over one another, some exposed cells die and peel away. New cells take their place from the growing ends that are attached to the bone surfaces on the two sides. In a well-hydrated cartilage, the rate of friction damage is minimal. In a dehydrated cartilage, the rate of "abrasive" damage is increased.

Low Back Pain

Spinal joints, intervertebral joints and their disc structures, are depended on different hydraulic properties of water stored in the disc core, as well as in the end plate cartilage covering the flat surfaces of the spinal vertebrae. In spinal vertebral joints water is not only a lubricant for the contact surfaces, it is held in the disc core within the intervertebral space and supports the compression weight of the upper body.

Approximately 75 percent of the weight of the upper part of the body is supported by water volume that is stored in the disc core and 25 percent is supported by the fibrous material around the disc. The principle in the design of all joints is for water to act as a lubricating agent, as well as to bear the force produced by weight, or tension produced by muscle action on the joint. Once dehydration sets in, all parts of the body begin to suffer. The intervertebral discs and their joints are the first in line. The fifth lumbar disc is affected in 96 percent of cases.

Chapter Eight

*We are enslaved by anything we do not consciously see.
We are freed by conscious perception.*
Vernon Howard

Cellular Oxygen Deficiency and Cancer

One of the most provocative theories regarding the cause of cancer was originally put forth by Nobel laureate Dr. Otto Warburg,[1] a German biochemist who won the Nobel Prize in 1931 for discovering that oxygen deficiency and cell fermentation are part of the cancer process.

According to Dr. Warburg's theory, when cells are deprived of oxygen they can revert to their "primitive" state and enter into glucose reactions, deriving energy not from oxygen as normal plant and animal cells do, but from the fermentation of sugar. Oxygen is dethroned in cancer cells and replaced by an energy-yielding reaction of the lowest forms, namely, a fermentation of glucose. Rapid reproduction of the cancer cells uses up large amounts of glucose, breaking it down into lactic acid. Lactic acid is a waste product that puts a strain on the body and causes an imbalance in the acid/alkaline ratio, or pH. As the acidity of the body rises it becomes even more difficult for the cells to use oxygen normally.

As cancer cells begin to multiply, forming a tumor, the liver must expend a considerable amount of energy converting the toxic lactic acid back to glucose. Also, most cancer cells can function only at a low pH (a very acidic state) because of the lactic acid they constantly produce. The combined effect of the tumor's metabolism is to tax the liver and acidify the body. Cancerous tumors may contain as much as ten times more lactic acid than healthy tissues.[2] Remember, cancer cells cannot exist in an oxygen-rich environment!

---

[1] Warburg, O. On the Origin of Cancer Cells. Science 123 (1956)
[2] Thomas, Gordon, Dr. Issels and His Revolutionary Cancer Treatment (New York: Peter H. Wyden, 1973), 137-138

An acid condition in the body can cause cells to become malignant. The acidity the intracellular fluids within the cell damages the cell nuclei which control cellular growth. Acidity in the extra cellular fluids kills the nerve cells that are connected with the brain reducing its ability to send proper messages to fight the dysfunctional cells (cancer). Hexagonal water's microclusters, which are made up of five to six water molecules, as a result of the electrolysis process,[3] are able to effectively enter the cells and remove the acid thus increasing the body's ability to fight the free-radicals.

---

[3] Small clusters mean the increased ability of water to dissolve elements as well as to be absorbed into your body.

Chapter Nine

> *"Of all the knowledge, the one most worth having is knowledge about health! The first requisite of a good life is to be a healthy person."*
> Herbert Spencer

So, What's in Your Water?

If we want to have safe drinking water and also avoid the potentially harmful effects of inhaling water pollutants or absorbing them through our skin, a first step is to understand the kinds of pollutants that may be in our water. Nuisance pollutants are those that cause discomfort or inconvenience. They can cause water to taste, smell, or look bad, and they can render soap and washing less effective.

The following are health-threatening pollutants:

- Pathogens
- Toxic minerals and metals
- Organic chemicals
- Radioactive substances
- Additives

Pathogens

Pathogens are harmful microorganisms such as bacteria, viruses and parasites. They can cause such diseases as typhoid, cholera, hepatitis, flu, and giardiasis. The most common bacteria are closely monitored in public water supplies. Private wells may be contaminated with bacteria. If the well is near a septic system, open to the air, or subject to chemical pollution or animal fecal matter.

Viruses are much smaller than bacteria and harder to detect. Viruses are very common in water. Although disinfected with chlorine (the method used by most public utilities) probably kills the majority of viruses in the water, no one knows for sure how many viruses remain potent.

The third type of pathogens commonly found in water is protozoan parasites. In people that have a suppressed immune system, these can be life threatening. Parasites can be present in public water supplies even though a water treatment plant is operating properly.

Toxic minerals

Toxic minerals are the harmful inorganic substances that are found in water supplies. They include metals as well as common minerals in the form of rock, sand, and clay. The inorganic minerals in water that are known to be harmful to our health in large quantities are:

- Aluminum
- Lead
- Barium
- Selenium
- Copper
- Fluoride
- Asbestos
- Nitrate
- Chromium
- Nitrite
- Arsenic
- Mercury
- Cadmium
- Silver

These toxic minerals and inorganic compounds occur naturally in water, and they also enter water from man-made sources. Some of them are more toxic than others. Cadmium, lead, and mercury have the greatest toxicity, and ingestion of even small amounts can be fatal. Asbestos is also present in tap water wherever asbestos-cement water pipes are used to deliver water to customers. Trace-minerals are organic absorbable and found in plants, algae and some supplements. These (chromium, copper, silver) are safe and beneficial to the body in the proper dosage. Inorganic minerals cannot be absorbed by the body, resulting in toxicity.

Organic Chemicals

Organic chemicals are substances that come directly from, or are manufactured from, plant or animal matter. Plastics, for example, are organic chemicals that are made from petroleum, which originally came from plant and animal matter. There are over 100,000 different manufactured, or synthetic, organic chemicals in commercial use today. In addition to the organic chemicals that have found their way into water supplies. New and dangerous one are created in the process of water treatment. Chlorine, which is added to essentially all U.S. public supplies, combines with organic compounds from decaying plant matter or sludge found in water system pipes, to form a category of toxic pollutants called trihalomethanes (THMs) that are carcinogens (substances that increase the risk of getting cancer).

Radioactive Substances

Radioactive substances in water fall into two categories: radioactive minerals and radioactive gases. Radioactive minerals can be either naturally occurring or man-made. When naturally occurring, their source is typically an area where mining is going on or has gone on in the past. Uranium mining produces radioactive runoff. There are other kinds of mines that enable radioactive minerals to enter water supplies. This is because mining exposes rock strata, most of which contain some amount of radioactive ore. Naturally occurring radioactive minerals also can enter water supplies through the operation of smelters and coal-fired electrical plants.

Man-made sources of radioactive minerals in the water are nuclear power plants, nuclear weapons facilities, radioactive materials disposal sites, and docks for nuclear-powered ships. Another source of radioactive pollution comes from hospitals all over the country, which are allowed to dump low-level radioactive wastes into sewers. Some of those radioactive wastes eventually find their way into water supplies.

Additives

Most public water treatment plants, from small community systems to larger urban waterworks, add things to water. These are added for a variety of reasons, ranging from disinfection to enhancing effectiveness of treatment to improving the water's aesthetic qualities.

The best-known additive is chlorine as mentioned earlier. According to studies conducted jointly at Harvard University and the Medical College of Wisconsin, the consumption of chlorinated drinking water accounts for 15 percent of all rectal cancers and 9 percent of all bladder cancers in the U.S. Further, people drinking chlorinated water over long periods of time have a 39 percent increase in their chances of contracting rectal cancer and a 21 percent increase in the risk of contracting bladder cancer.[4]

Water fluoridation

Fluoride, a poison second in toxicity only to arsenic, has routinely been added to public drinking water and toothpaste since the 1950s, despite mounting evidence of its health hazards. According to the scientific research, fluoride consumption creates multiple hazards with respect to cancer. Fluoride can actually produce cancer, transforming normal human cells into cancerous ones, even at concentrations of only 1 ppm (parts per million), the official "safe" dosage set by the U.S. Public Health Service for drinking water.

Flocculants

In addition to chlorine, and sometimes fluorine (a component of fluoride), water treatment plants often add several other substances to water to improve the efficiency of the treatment. Flocculants are substances added to water to make the particles in it clump together for more efficient removal by filtering.

Some of the most commonly used flocculants, called polyelectrolytes, have been banned in several other countries because some of their constituents are known to cause genetic mutations. The EPA classifies some of these flocculants as probable human carcinogens.

---

[4] Diamond, J. Cowden, W. Cancer Diagnosis, Alternative Publ. 2003

Chapter Ten

"Only I can change my life. No one else can do it for me."
Carol Burnett

Sports Drinks and Bottled Water

Recently, there has been introduced to the market, a flurry of sport drinks, mixes, and electrolyte supplements. The marketing goals appear to be focused on rehydration and increased sports performance. Certain preservatives, artificial flavors and colored dyes, aspartame, and sugar may add to the visual or taste appeal of the drink, but may not be user-friendly to the body.

While most companies producing the products seem to embrace the value of electrolytes, they may not have delivered the proper complement of trace-minerals for formation and absorption. For example, Boron is a necessary trace element needed for cellular absorption of other nutrients. Since most sports drinks contain only sodium and potassium rather than the proper complement of multi-minerals, they are unable to create the proper reaction to make electrolytes that are needed to keep the body's electrical system charged.

In addition to its usefulness after exercise to replenish glycogen stores, sugar (fructose, dextrose, glucose, high fructose corn syrup, maltodextrin) is usually added as a carbohydrate to boost energy levels. While this may stimulate the body momentarily, minutes later the glycemic roller coaster sets in with associated compromise in body function. Different studies reveal that sugar actually diffuses the body's ability to maintain muscle strength; therefore, it does not seem wise to use it when periods of strength are required. Sugar also creates cravings that generate a desire for more sweet drinks. In high quantities it also has been linked to diabetes. As blood glucose levels increase, people with diabetes are more at risk for heart disease. Besides sugared drinks, there are other ways to get carbohydrates, such as energy bars, and the complex carbohydrates found in apples, grapes, or peanuts. Furthermore, studies show that it may be the complex carbohydrates that support strength and endurance, rather than simple carbohydrates. As for other aspects of water, there can be a wide variation in the quality of bottled water from one type or brand to another.

Among the many weaknesses of the FDA (Food and Drug Administration) regulation is the fact that the FDA exempts intrastate bottled water (bottled water not sold outside the state where it originates) from regulation, even though 75 percent of all bottled water sold in the United States is intrastate. Seltzer, other carbonated waters, and flavored waters are also exempted. The FDA requires testing of bottled water less frequently than is required by the EPA (Environmental Protection Agency) for tap water and if a particular bottled water exceeds the limits for any pollutants, that water can still be legally sold.

Plastic Water Bottles

When water is placed in soft plastic bottles, it tends to leach out any chemicals in the plastic that are loosely bonded. These chemicals then enter the water in miniscule amounts. The longer water remains in a plastic bottle and the higher its temperature, the greater the chance of chemicals entering the water. For example, leaving a plastic water bottle in the car during the warm weather (and as the temperature rises in the car), the chemicals from the plastic bottle leach into the water, especially if you reuse these bottles. Most plastic bottles are for one time use. No guarantees are made for the integrity of the chemical bonding for multiple uses.

Some studies have shown a link between chemicals leached from plastic water bottles and disorders of the immune system. Recently the FDA has been asked to review the safety of food products that contain bisphenol-A, or BPA, a hormone-disrupting chemical most commonly used in the linings of polycarbonate water bottles, specifically those marked with a #7 inside the recycled symbol on the bottom of the container. We highly recommend consumers use either glass or stainless steel bottles. This also helps to reduce landfill waste. Electrolyte products are available to put in the refillable water bottles so you can make your own sports drink and control your intake of sugars. According to Nina Anderson, SPN, "sweetened sports drinks contribute to the obesity epidemic in the USA. Most of them also contain only sodium and potassium, which do not make effective electrolytes. You need in addition trace amounts of selenium, boron, copper, manganese, zinc, cobalt, silica, iodine and chromium to properly rehydrate the body."[5]

---

[5] Anderson, Nina, Analyzing Sports Drinks, 2002, Safe Goods, Sheffield, MA,

Chapter Eleven

"Nothing can bring you peace but yourself."
Ralph Waldo Emerson

What in the World is Hexagonal Water?

Hexagonal water is a specific arrangement of individual water molecules where six water (H_2O) units consistently link to form a ring-like structure. This unique arrangement is the basis of a more complex crystalline network that is formed when numerous hexagonal units join together. In other words, hexagonal water is a liquid crystal.

All water contains a certain percentage of hexagonal units, but the percentage of hexagonal units depends on certain conditions, including the energetic influences that water is exposed to. For example: chlorine, fluoride and many pollutants typically found in municipal water sources reduce the number of hexagonal units. Tap water typically has a very low percentage of hexagonal structures. On the other hand, there are a number of places throughout the world where the water has a high concentration of hexagonal structures. Many of these places are known as "healing springs." Other water sources are known for producing inhabitants who drink that water and live long and disease-free lives.

According to Dr. Mu Shik Jhon,[6] bulk water at 50 degrees Fahrenheit is 22 percent hexagonally structured. Other factors that influence hexagonal structure are temperature, structure-making minerals (sodium, lithium), and/or the presence of a weak magnetic field, electric or vibrational fields.

The difference between normal water (a structural conglomerate) and hexagonally structured water (an organized matrix) is similar to the difference between a piece of quartz and a quartz crystal. Although they are chemically the same,

---

[6] Jhon, M. The Water Puzzle and the Hexagonal Key, Uplifting Press 2004

quartz is a random organization of molecules. It has an almost opaque appearance. On the other hand, the molecules in a quartz crystal are organized in perfect geometric symmetry. Quartz crystals are clear. They have special properties which non-crystalline quartz does not possess. Computer chips and quartz watches rely on these unique properties, which are a function of the organization of the molecules in the crystalline form.

Hexagonal water is able to carry signals and transfer information with greater efficiency because of its high degree of organization. This organization is also responsible for a higher energy state that may be the key to rapid hydration, enhanced energy, protein and DNA stability, and the enhancement of numerous metabolic functions.

A majority of the water on the surface of the planet is a mixture of hexagonal units separated by other structural units and free water molecules. Even though water has a high-energy potential compared to other liquids, it is no match for the energetic potential of hexagonal water. When water molecules join to form hexamers, greater structural stability is created and the resulting water has the potential to hold more energy. As hexamers join to form the crystalline matrix, the energy is additive – just like increasing the voltage by adding batteries in series – the greater the hexagonal structuring in the water network, the greater the potential energy.

Hexagonal water and aging

When we are born, our bodies are more than 90 percent water (by weight), but the time we are in our twenties the amount of water is reduced to an average of 70 percent. When we are sixty or older, the total water content of our bodies is less than 50 percent.

As we age, the movement of water within our bodies also slows down, resulting in a reduced amount of water within the cells (cells actually wither just like a raisin). Since cells function best when 60 per cent of the total body's water is inside the cells, reduced water movement and a reduced amount of water inside the cells has been correlated with age.

Hexagonal water hydrates the cellular environment of the body more rapidly while delivering nutrients and removing wastes more efficiently. This would naturally influence the aging process. A recent study, using magnetic resonance imaging (MRI), tested the hypothesis that aging was related to structural changes in intracellular water. The structure of the cell water components of four generations within the same genetic family was analyzed. The conclusion was that age was, in fact, related to structural changes in the water surrounding biological macromolecules, and that the state of the water in the body was closely related to the aging mechanism. Getting hexagonal water into the cells of our bodies will be one of the most important things we do to prevent premature aging.[7]

Dehydration – the Lack of Cellular Water

As mentioned previously, dehydration is a condition that occurs when a person loses more fluid than they take in. However, the problem is not just a lack of water, it is a lack of cellular water! If the water we drink is prevented from entering cells we can drink water all day long and still be dehydrated.

When there is insufficient water inside the cells every function suffers and the body must operate from a level of crisis management. With a lack of cellular water, organs must compete for vital fluids – balance (homeostasis) gives way to disharmony and disease.

Remember, water is the body's main source of energy. Dr. Batmanghelidj, author of Your Body's Many Cries for Water, states, "The flow of water through the cell membrane provides electrical energy much like the turbines in a hydroelectric plant. As water rushes into the cells it creates the necessary electrical energy, tops off cellular reserves, then leaves the body taking with it the waste products from each cell."[8] Dr. Jhon, author of *The Water Puzzle and the*

---

[7] Katayama, S., "Aging Mechanism Associated with a Function of Biowater," Physiol Chem Phys and Med. NMR 24:43-50. 199
[8] Batmanghelidj, F., *Your Body's Many Cries for Water*, Global Health Solutions, 1992

Hexagonal Key, explains that hexagonal water actually has the capacity to hold more energy than normal water because of its structure and 100 percent hexagonally structured water has a huge capacity to store energy which can be released immediately when it is utilized by living organisms.[9]

Only when there is sufficient water do we have ample and ongoing energy – especially as we age. The consumption of hexagonal water enhances the amount of electrical energy available in the body, improves cellular water environment, and cellular efficiency. Drinking hexagonal water is one of the easiest ways to overcome chronic dehydration and to protect our body from disease and premature aging.

Because aging is also correlated with a loss of water the skin is a good indicator of age. Aging and dehydration result in thin, wrinkled skin, which has lost its resiliency. Try this test: Gently pinch the skin on the back of your hand between the thumb and forefinger for six seconds. Then count how many seconds it takes for the skin to flatten out again. The length of time it takes can be correlated with age, dehydration, and skin health. Generally, those between the ages of 45 and 50 have a return-response time under 6 seconds, but by the age of 60, the amount of time it takes for the skin to return to its original position is double or triple (10-15 seconds), and by the age of 70, the response time is typically 35 to 40 seconds.

The lack of resiliency in older skin is due to a loss of water. As we age, the thirst mechanism declines and water is lost from many areas of the body. The structure of the water within our bodies also deteriorates with age making it less efficient and less mobile. The aging process is literally a withering of the tissues throughout the body – visibly reflected in the skin.

Hexagonal water, because of its organization, rehydrates the body much more rapidly than normal water. It moves into the cells almost immediately shown by Live Blood Analysis. This is one reason why so many individuals notice an improvement in the condition of their skin when they drink hexagonal water.

---

[9] Jhon, M.S., *The Water Puzzle and the Hexagonal Key*, Uplifting Press, 2004

Many notice softer skin within days. Improvements in acne, dry skin and other conditions are common. They are an indication of the internal face lift that is reflected in the skin "a face lift from the inside out".

As we are beginning to discover, one of the biggest factors in the quality of the water we drink is molecular structure. Not only does hexagonal water have the capacity to hold more energy, but also because of its organization it is actually more efficient water augmenting everything that water does in the human body. Drinking hexagonal water can play a remarkable role when it comes to reducing the effects of environmental stress on our bodies.

Hexagonal water moves within biological organisms with greater ease supporting cellular processes and cellular communication. It is also capable of taking nutrients more rapidly into the bloodstream. Once there a greater content of water in the blood it separates blood cells and provides more surface area for nutrient and oxygen exchange. Not only does hexagonal water move into the cells more easily, it also moves out of the cells more rapidly carrying toxins and metabolic waste. Regular and ongoing consumption of hexagonal water replaces unorganized water with hexagonal water increasing energy at the cellular level, improving nutrient absorption, enhancing detoxification, and reducing the effects of aging.

To maintain proper hydration it is recommended that we need to consume a minimum of 2 liters (8 glasses/64 oz.) of hexagonal water a day. Athletes need to consume 16 ounces 30 minutes before exercise. Then, depending on temperature and duration of exercise, they need to consume 4 to 12 ounces every thirty minutes.

During strenuous activity blood volume decreases. This is due to an overall reduction in body water (blood is between 85-94 percent water). Reduced blood volume diminishes the oxygen to the muscles and has a subsequent effect on endurance and performance. Hexagonal water increases blood volume, improves blood flow and increases endurance.

Following the consumption of hexagonal water, live blood analysis illustrates the rapid reduction in agglutination (clumping) of red blood cells (representing the capacity for greater oxygen uptake and more efficient nutrient utilization). It also represents an improved ability to remove cellular waste. A recent test[10] showed that mice that consumed hexagonal water for thirty days nearly doubled their exercise time and had higher levels of glycogen (primary source of fuel during exercise) storage in the liver.

Surface Tension

One of the most easily measured differences between hexagonally-structured and bulk water is the surface tension. The reason that water "beads up" on any non-polar surface such as glass, is due to the high degree of surface tension (the tendency of the molecules to be tightly held together).

Most filtered and bottled water has a surface tension above 70 dynes/cm. Water from any fresh mountain stream has been measured below 65 dynes/cm. Some hexagonal water products claim a surface tension far below this level, making it "wetter." Lower surface tension naturally augments nutrient absorption and cellular cleansing. Many people state that hexagonal water actually tastes smoother and wetter, and many athletes have noticed that hexagonal water does not stay in their stomach as long moving noticeable quicker into the cellular components of their bodies.

Water's Memory

There is a strong indication that water has the capacity to maintain the energy/frequency of a substance placed in it – even after the substance is removed. Processing with electric fields enhances and even stabilizes molecular structural changes, which can last for extended periods of time. It is also possible for water that has been hexagonal-structured at one time, to "remember" and assume the structure once inside the body facilitating maximum absorption.

---

[10] Chen, D., et al, "Enhancement of swimming endurance by oral administration of clustered water." J. Internat. Soc. of Sports Nutr. (2005) 2(1): 1-30 Poster #42

Chapter Twelve

Take care of your body with steadfast fidelity. The soul must see through these eyes alone, and if they are dim, the whole world is clouded."
Johann Wolfgang Von Goethe

The Kangen™ Water Experience

The word Kangen™ means, "return to origin" in Japanese. In order to be called Kangen™, water must be alkaline, micro-clustered (hexagonal structure), pure, and have a high negative ORP (oxidation-reduction potential).

ORP is a measure of antioxidant power and is measured in millivolts (mV). It measures the presence of free electrons. A negative ORP means that a substance can donate free electrons, making it an antioxidant. A positive ORP means that a substance is taking electrons, making it a free radical or pro-oxidant.

Oxidation occurs when the oxygen molecule loses an electron and it becomes a free radical that begins to search for any molecule that might have an extra electron. Oxidation is how our bodies age resulting in wrinkles, degeneration of organs, bones, muscles, tendons, and cellular membranes. A reducing agent is simply something that inhibits or slows the process of oxidation.

The ORP of most tap water in the USA is between +200 to +600mV and so is an oxidizing agent. High pH ionized water demonstrates a negative (-)ORP and so is a reducing agent or "antioxidant". Most bottled waters are very acidic (low pH) and also have higher ORP's (over +400mV).

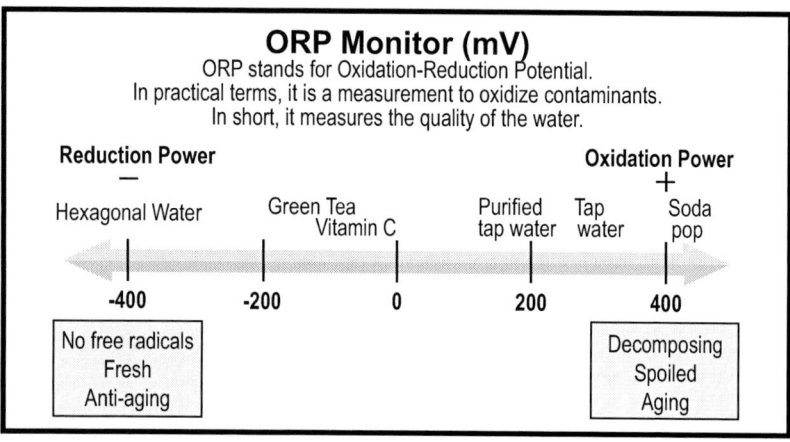

Hexagonal Kangen™ water, with an abundance of hydroxyl ions (OH-), provides extra electrons that neutralize destructive free radicals circulating throughout the body. Hexagonal Kangen™ water carries a high negative ORP when it is produced. Dr. Hayashi, Director of the Water Institute in Tokyo, Japan, states, "When taken internally the reduced ionized water with redox potential or ORP, is ORP of -250 to -350mV readily donates its electrons to oddball oxygen radicals and blocks the interaction of the active oxygen with normal molecules."

As previously mentioned, proper pH is an important factor in good health. If any substance changes from pH 7 to pH 8 it has become ten times more alkaline. Conversely, if it has changes from neutral pH 7 to pH 6 it is ten times more acidic. For example, soda pop at pH 2.5 is almost 50,000 times more acidic than neutral water, and needs 32 glasses of neutral (pH 7) water to counteract the consumption of one glass of soda. Please understand from this that our blood pH can be affected at any time of the day by events, food, drink, stress, pollution, and exercise.

Hexagonal Kangen™ water is alkaline, able to neutralize and balance a chronic over-acid state. The body draws upon alkaline minerals stored in the bones and tissues to buffer the over-acid state. Hexagonal Kangen™ water helps the body preserve and maintain its calcium, magnesium, and potassium reserves by providing ionic minerals and negative hydroxyl ions to buffer excess acids.

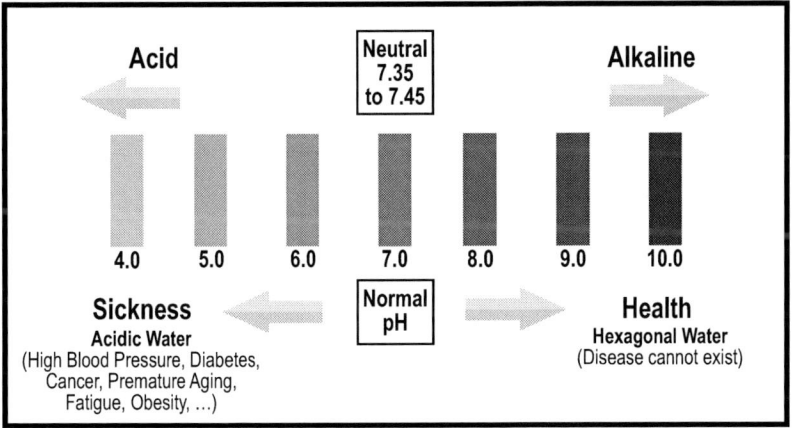

pH and ORP alteration is a highly variable and depends on various factors:
- Electrolysis is a process where electricity is passed through electrodes composed of precious metals with the ability to attract ions that conduct electricity. The ions that are naturally present in water are then concentrated into clusters of positive and negatively charged ions and separated by a membrane. This process restructures the original water clusters into smaller hexagonal clusters that are either positively or negatively charged. This simultaneously creates both alkaline (8.5 - 9.5 pH) water for drinking, and acidic (4.5 - 5.5) pH water, ionized for topical use.
- Acidic water is also known as electro-oxidizing water and has unique characteristic including high positive ORP, low pH, and a high concentration of dissolved chloride and oxygen. In Japanese hospitals electro-oxidizing water is used to treat skin ulcers, sterilize wounds and keep hospitals clear of infectious bacteria and viruses.

True hexagonal Kangen™ water depends on two factors: the size or surface area of the electrolysis plates and the amount of electrical power used to accomplish the electrolysis process. While many water ionizers produce "alkaline" water, when tested under normal operating conditions, the pH and ORP measurements of water produced by these ionizers are inconsistent due to the use of small platinum coating plates (small plates heat up more quickly, thus causing the alkalinity to drop off sharply) and low power (electricity is the power that splits the water molecule and produces the desirable hexagonal molecular structure, more power is definitely better).[11]

Stomach Acid and Kangen™ Water

According to many experts, the most important function of hexagonal Kangen™ water is to increase bicarbonates in the blood. As we age, we lose bicarbonates, which buffer or neutralize acids.[12] Alkalizing the body means increasing the number of bicarbonate buffers available to the interstitial fluids surrounding the cells. The blood pH does not change, but the ability of our body to neutralize acid increases.

When and How Much

One of the best times to drink hexagonal Kangen™ water is first thing in the morning. After six to eight hours without water, the body's reserves need to be replenished. With one eight-ounce glass of hexagonal Kangen™ water upon arising, the digestive tract is primed for breakfast. This helps to prevent water rationing and all its complication.

A good habit is to drink eight ounces of hexagonal Kangen™ water on an empty stomach 15 minutes before eating, since hydrochloric acid is necessary to digest proteins. When empty, the stomach pH value may be low (acidic), and the amount (volume) of hydrochloric acid in the stomach is

---

[11] McCauley, B., *The Miraculous Properties of Ionized Water*, Spartan Enterprises, 2006

[12] Frasetto, L. Journal of Gerontology: Biological Sciences, 1996, Vol. 51A, No. 1, B91-B99

small. Also, as we age the hydrochloric acid in our stomach becomes normally less. Therefore, drinking 9.5 pH hexagonal Kangen™ water will raise the stomach pH relatively high. The stomach then naturally produces more hydrochloric acid to return its pH to normal (4.0 pH), which results in more bicarbonates entering the bloodstream.

Drinking before every meal has other advantages like helping the body to distinguish between thirst and hunger. Many people do not eat as much when they begin with a glass of hexagonal Kangen™ water. When water is consumed before a meal we also tend to chew more completely, rather than washing food down. Finally, it is a good idea to drink another eight ounces of water two to three hours after each meal. In this way, water is continually being consumed throughout the day.

Hexagonal Kangen™ water is perfect when taken with nutritional supplements. It aids in a more complete assimilation of the nutrients. For the same reason, medication should not be taken with hexagonal Kangen™ water. It may have a more potent effect and be too strong. It has been recommended that any medication be taken either an hour before or an hour after drinking hexagonal Kangen™ water. It is also a good idea to work with a health practitioner when consuming hexagonal Kangen™ water, especially if you are taking prescription medications. Some individuals have been able to reduce or even eliminate certain medications.

Healing Crisis

A healing crisis is when the body's natural defense systems are waging war on the illness itself and is trying to purge the illness from the body. People whose systems are quite toxic may go through a healing crises. During this time, symptoms may worsen. However, this healing crises will normally only last a few short days, and when over the body heals very rapidly. Improvements in health will be extremely noticeable. The healing crisis can be uncomfortable but once it has passed people have been astounded at how well they begin to feel. In all cases drinking hexagonal Kangen™ water has produced results that have been observed in a time period ranging from a few days to as many as 12 weeks, normally averaging four to six weeks.

Chapter Thirteen

What People Are Saying About Kangen™ Water

Because of Kangen™ water's ability to rejuvenate the body, practitioners and their patients who use it have reported numerous benefits: Some reports include the ability to:

- Reduce chronic pain
- Release excess body fat and stored toxins
- Normalize blood pressure
- Support healthy colon function
- Normalize blood sugar and insulin
- Resolve urinary tract infections
- Relieve asthma and chronic respiratory infections
- Stop abnormal gastrointestinal putrefaction
- Improve wound healing
- Reduce proliferation of candida

Many people are achieving wondrous results using Kangen™ water. There are devices out in the market place claiming to be great ionizer systems, but the Kangen™ system is different from all of them because it was designed with its specific purpose already determined. It is based solidly on medical research. The device utilizes the technology of Kangen™ that is rapidly becoming state of the art.

Consider, for example, the following from Dr. Dave Carpenter, N.D., well known for his expertise on the benefits of hexagonal water:

> "In the early 1990's I had the opportunity to spend some time in Japanese hospitals where I observed the treatment of terrible cases of eczema, psoriasis, diabetic ulcers and even gangrene treated with special water. It seemed to me that this water was doing more for the

people suffering from these conditions than any other form of treatment I was aware. I came home convinced that I needed this amazing water the Japanese called hexagonal water to use with my patients

"Hexagonal water is only found in nature in the high mountains where it is formed by glacier ice or snow melt. This creates water that is a 6-sided or hexagonal structure and approximately 1/3 the size of most water. As this hexagonal water flows down out of the mountains into rivers and streams and pipes, holding tanks and bottles the action of the sun shining on this water turns it into a pentagonal shape (5 sided) and the molecules clump in groups of 15 to 20 molecules. This water is what most of us drink and it is not readily absorbed and utilized by the body. Let me give you an example. If you drink 20 to 30 ounces of "normal" water (pentagonal structured water) at one time it will feel like your stomach is like a water balloon, with water sloshing around for some time because the body cannot absorb it quickly and easily. Drinking the same amount of hexagonal water will not produce that same feeling in the stomach for any length of time because it absorbs much more readily.

"In July of 2006 I was introduced to a Japanese made ionizer called the SD 501 produced by company named Enagic. I could tell a difference in just drinking the water compared to the water produced by other machines. I also put a scoop of a green drink powder I like to take in the water and noticed that in this Kangen™ water the powder stayed in solution rather than ended up on the bottom of the bottle over time. This had never happened in water produced by any of the other ionizers that I'd used. I was cautiously hopeful that I had found a machine that really could produce water that would make the differences I'd been hoping for all these years. I began sharing the water with patients. For the first time they were coming back to get more water and telling me of all of the health miracles they were experiencing. Things like less depression, better sleep, more energy, reduced pain and inflammation, reduced headaches, better mental clarity, and many more amazing health improvements. Almost everyone came back two or three times per week to get more water. Soon these folks were so excited that they were telling their friends to get water at our clinic or purchase their own machines."

-Dr. David Carpenter

Reports from Dr. Carpenter's case studies:

"Linda E. from Idaho had a sinus infection in March of 2007. She was taken off all dairy and put on Kangen water daily along with GSE for infection. The infection cleared up in a few days and she also lost 10 pounds. She also had high cholesterol, high blood sugar and joint pain and her M.D. wanted her to lose at least 50 pounds. She continued to drink 4 to 5 quarts of Kangen water daily and followed an 80/20 diet (80% alkaline/20% acidic foods) and in 12 months lost 117 pounds total with no saggy baggy skin."

"Amy II. from Idaho was diagnosed with Crohn's disease seven years ago. During the past seven years she had experienced pain after eating, diarrhea, weight loss, symptoms of malnutrition, blurry eyesight, memory loss, swollen joints, skin conditions, anemia, compromised immune function and many other issues. Her diet was restricted to a bland, fiberless diet and most days she ate very little because eating caused so much discomfort. She consulted with GI doctors, family practitioners, internists, rheumatologists, urologists, emergency room doctors and everyone else that may have an idea. She tried various pharmaceuticals, tried many diets, read every book she could find on Crohn's disease and tried a wide assortment of herbals treatments as well.

Nothing really worked for her and she ended up having a bowel resection (emergency) in June of 2006. Things didn't improve. In June of 2007 she went to Dr. Carpenter and I suggested starting with the Kangen™ water. She used the 8.5 pH water for 30 days before moving up to the 9.0 pH water. Over six to eight weeks most of her symptoms slowly disappeared. After eight months of drinking the water she is eating again, gaining weight back, and have energy to do most things she wants to do. She is eating raw vegetables, corn on the cob, popcorn and other foods that she had not eaten in seven years."

"Ivan C. from Missouri had struggled with elevated cholesterol for years and had been on several prescription medications to help control that. Blood tests on 10/3/07 showed Cholesterol at 235 with Triglycerides at 296, HDL at 48 and LDL at 127.8. He stopped drinking soda's and began drinking Kangen™ water in December of 2007 and blood tests performed on 2/5/08 revealed total cholesterol of 176, triglycerides of 139, HDL at 52 and LDL at 96.2."

What other people have reported about Kangen™ *water:*

"For years I have suffered off and on with arthritis. In the last several months it has gotten worse. The doctors suggested I have knee replacement surgery. A friend suggested I start drinking hexagonal Kangen™ water daily. Gradually, I started noticing a change. My hands became more flexible. In fact I was able to make a fist without any pain. My knees were becoming pain free. I am able to walk around without using a cane. Bless the person who introduced me to Kangen™ water."

-Lee E., New Mexico

"I have been drinking Kangen™ water for less than a year. I have experienced many grateful effects. I have a family history of high cholesterol and high blood pressure. My total cholesterol was 265 before drinking the water. My latest blood test showed my cholesterol number dropped 75 points. My blood pressure is now within the normal range. I truly believe the numbers changed totally due to drinking Kangen™ water, as I did not make any other changes, even though my doctor wanted me to take medication."

-Sarah K., California

"For many years, I have had doctors tell me that my Fibromyalgia symptoms were all in my head. I tried many remedies to alleviate my pain and symptoms and did not find anything that would help. I started drinking hexagonal Kangen™ water about six months ago. After a few weeks of drinking the water, my pain subsided. It even is helping me with other conditions that have baffled me. I am totally pain free and very grateful for being introduced to Kangen™ water."

-Pat. M., Texas

Create A Miracle

Resources

Kangen™ Water

Drinking fresh hexagonal Kangen™ water gives the body more anti-oxidant power and deep hydration. Owning a unit also makes it possible to drink as much pure hexagonal Kangen™ water as your body desires every day with no waste of plastic bottles or concern about drinking plastic-contaminated water. And the cost is considerably less over the life of the generator than bottles or designed water. Owning a unit also allows you to benefit from the other types of water that can be produced.

"Change Your Water ... Change Your Life"
Kangen™ Water Experience

For more information contact:

Mort Farina
Town Center Compounding Pharmacy
Palm Desert CA 92260
310-880-2537 (cell)

Bibliography

Anderson, N. and Peiper, H., *The Secrets of Staying Young*, Safe Goods, Sheffield, MA 2008

Anderson, N., *Analyzing Sports Drinks*, Safe Goods, Sheffield MA, 2002

Batmanghelidj, F., *Your Body's Many Cries for Water*, Global Health Solutions, 1997

Bell, R. and Peiper, H., *The ADD & ADHD Diet*, Safe Goods, Sheffield, MA 2007

Diamond, J. and Cowden, W., *Cancer Diagnosis*, Alternative Medicine, 2000

Emoto, M., *The True Power of Water*, Beyond Words, 2005

Ingram, C., *The Drinking Water Book*, Celestial Arts, 2006

Jhon, M. S., *The Water Puzzle and the Hexagonal Key*, Uplifting Press, 2004

Tunsky, G., *The Battle for Health is over pH*, Crusador Enterprises, 2007

About The Author

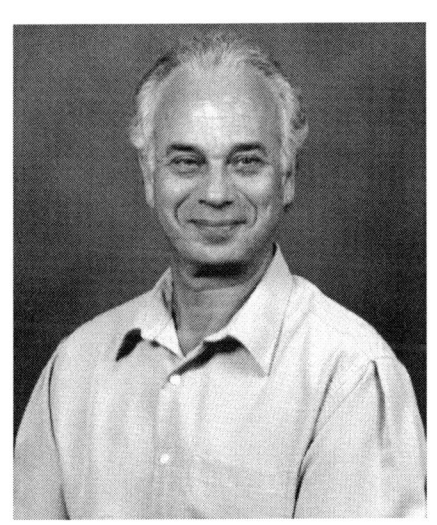

Dr. Howard Peiper, **N.D.**
nominated for a Pulitzer Prize, has written/co-authored many books on nutrition and natural health including the best-seller, The A.D.D. and A.D.H.D. Diet.

Notes

Notes

other books by
ATN/Safe Goods Publishing

The ADD and ADHD Diet Expanded	$ 10.95 US
ADD, The Natural Approach	5.95 US
Testosterone is your Friend	8.95 US
Eye Care Naturally	8.95 US
The Natural Prostate Cure	6.95 US
The Minerals You Need	4.95 US
The Smart Brain Train	7.95 US
New Hope for Serious Diseases	7.95 US
What is Beta Glucan?	4.95 US
Cancer Disarmed Expanded	7.95 US
The Vertical System	9.95 US
Overcoming Senior Moments Expanded	9.95 US
Crissy the CowPot Gets Her Wish!	9.95 US
Lower Cholesterol without Drugs	6.95 US
The Secrets of Staying Young	11.95 US
Worse Than Global Warming	9.95 US
2012 Airborne Prophesy	16.95 US
The Natural Diabetes Cure	8.95 US
Rx for Computer Eyes	8.95 US
Kids First: Health with No Interference	16.95 US

For a complete listing of books
visit our web site:
www.longlifecatalogs.com
to order or for a free catalog call
(888) 628-8731